Coconut oil

A comprehensive knowledge on how coconut oil is being extracted for our daily skin care

Dr Walt wade

Contents

chapter1

introduction to coconut oil

Coconut oil is a versatile, nutrient-rich oil that has become increasingly popular in recent years. It is commonly used as a cooking oil and in beauty products, but its benefits extend far beyond these uses. In this article, we will delve into the origins, properties, and uses of coconut oil, providing a comprehensive introduction to this much-loved oil. Origin and Properties of Coconut Oil Coconut oil is extracted from the kernel or meat of mature coconuts, which are the fruit of the coconut palm tree (Cocos nucifera). The trees are grown in tropical regions, primarily in Asia, Africa, and Latin America. The oil is traditionally extracted by grating and pressing the coconut meat, which yields a milky white substance. This substance is then left to stand until the oil separates from the water and solid particles. Coconut oil has a unique chemical composition, comprising mainly of saturated fats (over 80%), with smaller amounts of monounsaturated and polyunsaturated fats. It also contains vitamins E and K and minerals such as iron, zinc, and calcium. The distinctive properties of coconut oil are due to its high concentration of medium-chain fatty acids, specifically lauric acid (about 50%). These medium-chain fatty acids are quickly absorbed by the body and are known for their anti-inflammatory and antimicrobial properties. Uses of

Coconut Oil In traditional medicine, coconut oil has been used for centuries for its healing properties, especially in Ayurvedic and traditional Chinese medicine. With its high nutrient profile, it has been considered a powerful therapeutic agent for a range of conditions. Today, it continues to be used in traditional medicine and also in modern Western medicine. Cooking: Coconut oil has a high smoke point, making it suitable for high-temperature cooking methods such as frying, baking, and roasting. Its unique flavor and aroma make it a popular choice for Asian and Caribbean dishes. Additionally, its high concentration of medium-chain fatty acids has been linked to weight loss and improved metabolism, making it a popular choice for those following a ketogenic or low-carb diet. Skin and Hair Care: Coconut oil is a common ingredient in many beauty and skincare products due to its nourishing and moisturizing properties. It is believed to have a protective effect on the skin, improving its barrier function and preventing moisture loss. Its antimicrobial properties also make it beneficial for acne-prone skin. In hair care, coconut oil is often used to condition and add shine to dry, damaged hair. Oral Health: Recent studies have shown that coconut oil can have a positive impact on oral health. Its medium-chain fatty acids help fight harmful bacteria in the mouth, reducing the risk of cavities and gum disease. Oil pulling, a traditional Ayurvedic practice of swishing coconut oil in the mouth, is gaining popularity as a natural oral hygiene method. Digestive Health: Coconut oil has been linked to improved digestive health, especially for those with inflammatory bowel diseases. Its anti-inflammatory properties can help reduce inflammation in the gut and improve digestive function. Additionally, the medium-chain fatty acids in coconut oil can be easily absorbed and utilized by the body for energy, making it beneficial for those with digestive disorders that may affect nutrient absorption. Other Uses: Coconut oil has many other practical uses beyond cooking and beauty. It is commonly used as a natural moisturizer for dry skin and has been found to be effective in treating eczema and other skin conditions. It can also be used as a natural lubricant, in oil pulling for overall oral health, and as a natural insect repellent. Its high smoke point also makes it ideal for oiling wooden cutting boards and preserving wood furniture. Types of Coconut Oil There are several types of coconut oil available on the market, each with its unique properties. Here are the three most common types: Virgin vs. Refined: Virgin coconut oil is extracted without the use of chemicals or heat, resulting in a pure, unrefined product. It has a distinct coconut flavor and aroma and retains all of its beneficial properties. On the other hand, refined coconut oil undergoes a process of bleaching, deodorizing, and refining, which removes the coconut flavor and aroma. This type of coconut oil is more suitable for high-temperature cooking and has a longer shelf life, but it may also have a lower nutrient profile compared to virgin coconut oil. Fractionated: Fractionated coconut oil is produced by removing the long-chain fatty acids to create an oil that remains liquid at room temperature. It does not have a coconut aroma and is often used in skincare and massage oils due to its ability to quickly absorb into the skin. However, it may not have the same beneficial properties as other types of coconut oil. Extra-Virgin: Extra-virgin coconut oil is a high-quality product that is made from fresh coconut meat, extracted without the use of heat or chemicals. It has a stronger coconut flavor and aroma compared to virgin coconut oil and is considered to have the most beneficial properties. Conclusion Coconut oil is a versatile and highly beneficial oil with a long history of use in traditional medicine. Its unique properties and nutrient profile make it a popular choice for both internal and external use. From cooking and skincare to oral hygiene and digestive health, coconut oil has a wide array of uses and benefits. With its growing popularity and availability, there's no doubt that coconut oil will continue to be a staple in many

chapter2

coconut oil for skin

First and foremost, coconut oil is an excellent moisturizer for the skin. It is composed of saturated fats, making it easily absorbed into the skin, resulting in a deep hydration. This is especially beneficial for those with dry skin, as it provides intense moisture without clogging pores or leaving a greasy residue. The lauric acid in coconut oil also has antimicrobial properties, helping to combat bacteria and fungi that can lead to skin infections. Regular use of coconut oil can result in soft, supple, and healthy-looking skin. In addition to its moisturizing properties, coconut oil can also act as a natural anti-aging remedy. It is rich in antioxidants, which help fight free radicals that can cause skin damage and premature aging. Coconut oil also contains vitamin E, known for its ability to promote skin cell regeneration. This means that it can help minimize the appearance of fine lines and wrinkles, giving the skin a more youthful and radiant glow. Another significant benefit of coconut oil for skin is its anti-inflammatory properties. It contains fatty acids, such as linoleic and oleic acid, which help to reduce inflammation in the skin. This makes it an excellent option for those with inflammatory skin conditions, such as eczema, psoriasis, and rosacea. The soothing nature of coconut oil can provide relief from itching, redness, and irritation, making it a natural and gentle alternative to harsh topical creams. Coconut oil is also a versatile product that can be used for various skin concerns. For example, its antibacterial properties make it an effective treatment for acne-prone skin. The lauric acid in coconut oil can help to reduce the bacteria that cause acne, resulting in a clearer complexion. It also has a low comedogenic rating, meaning that it is less likely to clog pores and cause breakouts. For those struggling with dry, cracked lips, coconut oil is a lifesaver. Its moisturizing properties can help heal and nourish dry, chapped lips, making them soft and smooth again. It can also act as a natural lip balm, providing a protective barrier against the elements. Furthermore, it is safe to ingest, making it an excellent option for those who want to avoid harmful chemicals found in many lip products. Aside from its topical application, consuming coconut oil can also benefit the skin. When consumed in moderation, it can improve overall skin health and appearance. As mentioned before, coconut oil is rich in antioxidants and fatty acids, making it a nourishing addition to one's diet. It can help fight inflammation and free radicals from within, resulting in radiant and healthy-looking skin. But it's not just the skin on our face that can benefit from coconut oil. It can also be used on the body, particularly in areas that are prone to dryness, such as the elbows and knees. Regular use of coconut oil on these areas can help soften and smoothen rough patches of skin, giving a more even appearance overall. Coconut oil also has the ability to strengthen the skin's barrier function. This is important as the skin's barrier is responsible for protecting against environmental stressors, such as UV rays, pollutants, and bacteria. When the skin's barrier is compromised, it can lead to skin issues such as dryness, sensitivity, and even accelerated aging. The fatty acids in coconut oil help to strengthen and repair this protective layer, keeping the skin healthy and resilient. Aside from its many skincare benefits, coconut oil is also a cost-effective option. It is readily accessible in most supermarkets and health stores, and a little goes a long way. This makes it a budget-friendly alternative to expensive skincare products, giving you the same if not better results. However, it is essential to note that not all coconut oil is created equal. When purchasing coconut oil for skincare, it is best to opt for organic, cold-pressed, and unrefined options. This ensures that the oil is free from harmful chemicals and retains its nutrients and beneficial properties. It is also best to patch test the oil before using it all over the body, as with any new product, to avoid any potential allergic reactions.

coconut oil for hair

The Benefits of Coconut Oil for Hair: 1. Nourishes and Moisturizes: Coconut oil is rich in fatty acids, which penetrate deep into the hair shaft and help to nourish and moisturize the hair. It is also known for its ability to retain moisture in the hair, making it an excellent natural remedy for dry and damaged hair. The unique molecular structure of coconut oil allows it to penetrate the hair shaft and provide nourishment from within, leaving the hair soft, shiny and healthy. 2. Prevents Hair Damage: One of the main causes of hair damage is protein loss, which can lead to dull, dry and brittle hair. Coconut oil is packed with fatty acids that can help to replenish the lost proteins in the hair, reducing the risk of further damage. Regular use of coconut oil can also help to protect the hair from heat and environmental damage, making it an ideal option for those who use styling tools and live in polluted areas. 3. Promotes Hair Growth and Thickness: Coconut oil contains lauric acid, which has been linked to hair growth and thickness. Lauric acid easily penetrates the hair follicles, nourishing them and promoting healthy hair growth. It also helps to reduce protein loss in the hair, which can lead to thicker and stronger strands. Regular use of coconut oil can result in thicker, fuller and healthier-looking hair. 4. Fights Dandruff and Scalp Issues: Coconut oil has natural anti-fungal and anti-bacterial properties, making it an effective treatment for dandruff and other scalp issues. It can help to soothe an itchy scalp and reduce inflammation, which are common symptoms of dandruff. The moisturizing properties of coconut oil can also help to combat dry scalp, adding shine and moisture to the hair while promoting a healthy scalp. 5. Acts as a Natural Hair Conditioner: Commercial hair conditioners are often filled with harmful chemicals that can do more harm than good to the hair. Coconut oil, on the other hand, is a natural and safe alternative that can be used as a hair conditioner. It can help to soften and detangle the hair, making it easier to manage and style. It also helps to seal the hair cuticles, locking in moisture and making the hair shinier and more lustrous. How to Use Coconut Oil for Hair: There are many ways to incorporate coconut oil into your hair care routine. Here are a few simple methods that you can try at home: 1. Pre-Shampoo Treatment: Before shampooing your hair, gently massage a small amount of coconut oil onto your scalp and throughout your hair. Leave it on for at least 30 minutes (or overnight for a deeper treatment), and then wash your hair as usual. This pre-shampoo treatment will help to nourish and moisturize your hair, making it more manageable and less prone to breakage. 2. Hot Oil Treatment: For an intensive and deep conditioning treatment, warm up a generous amount of coconut oil and apply it to your hair and scalp. Wrap your hair in a towel or shower cap and leave it on for at least 30 minutes (or overnight). The heat will help the oil to penetrate deep into the hair shaft, providing maximum nourishment and hydration. Afterward, wash your hair as usual. 3. Leave-in Conditioner: If you have dry, curly or frizzy hair, using coconut oil as a leave-in conditioner can do wonders. After washing your hair, apply a small amount of coconut oil to the ends of your hair and work your way up. This will help to moisturize and define your curls, leaving your hair soft and hydrated. 4. Hair Mask: Mixing coconut oil with other natural ingredients, such as honey, avocado or egg, can create a powerful hair mask that can address specific hair concerns. For example, mixing coconut oil with honey can provide shine and moisture, while adding avocado can help to repair and strengthen damaged hair. Coconut oil can also be used as a styling product, providing a natural and healthy alternative to traditional hair gels and serums. A pea-sized amount of coconut oil can be used to tame flyaways and add shine to the hair, without weighing it down or leaving any greasy residue.

chapter3

coconut oil capsules

Coconut oil is extracted from the flesh of mature coconuts and is composed of medium-chain fatty acids (MCFAs) such as lauric acid, caprylic acid, and capric acid. These fatty acids are known to have numerous health benefits, making coconut oil a prized ingredient in natural health and beauty products. With the advent of coconut oil capsules, it has become even more convenient to reap the benefits of this superfood. One of the main reasons for the popularity of coconut oil capsules is its ease of use. The capsules come in a small, easy-to-swallow form, making it convenient for people to consume them on the go. Unlike oils, which can be messy and difficult to ingest, the capsules provide a neat and convenient way to consume coconut oil without any hassle. They are also odorless and have a neutral taste, making them suitable for people who do not like the flavor of coconut oil. There are various health benefits associated with coconut oil, and consuming it in a capsule form makes it easier to incorporate it into one's daily routine. The MCFAs found in coconut oil are known to have antiviral, antifungal, and antibacterial properties, making it a potent immune booster. Studies have shown that consuming coconut oil capsules can help in fighting off infections and diseases caused by harmful microorganisms. The medium-chain fatty acids in coconut oil are also known to help with weight loss. These fatty acids are easily digested and can be used as a source of instant energy. Consuming coconut oil capsules can help in speeding up the metabolism, promoting fat burning, and reducing appetite, leading to weight loss. Additionally, coconut oil contains healthy saturated fats that can keep one feeling full for longer, reducing the desire to snack on unhealthy foods. Coconut oil capsules are also gaining popularity for their potential to improve brain function. The MCFAs in coconut oil can provide an extra source of energy for the brain and have been linked to improved cognitive function, especially in people with Alzheimer's disease. A study found that consuming coconut oil capsules daily helped improve memory and brain function in Alzheimer's patients. They are also believed to have a positive effect on other neurological disorders such as Parkinson's disease and epilepsy, making it a promising natural remedy for these conditions. Another benefit of coconut oil capsules is their potential to improve heart health. The MCFAs in coconut oil have been shown to raise the levels of good cholesterol (HDL) and lower the levels of bad cholesterol (LDL). This can help in reducing the risk of heart disease and stroke. Coconut oil capsules are also known to have anti-inflammatory properties, which can benefit those suffering from heart disease or other chronic inflammatory conditions.

Coconut oil capsules are also becoming popular for their benefits on skin and hair health. The MCFAs in coconut oil have been proven to have moisturizing and nourishing properties when applied topically. In capsule form, coconut oil can help improve skin hydration, reduce signs of aging, and even promote hair growth. Consuming coconut oil capsules regularly can help one achieve healthier, glowing skin and luscious hair. One of the key reasons why people opt for coconut oil capsules is their potency and effectiveness. Unlike other supplements, which may contain fillers and artificial ingredients, coconut oil capsules are made from 100% pure coconut oil. This ensures that one is getting the full benefits of the oil without any potentially harmful additives. Additionally, coconut oil capsules are easy to digest, making it suitable for those with sensitive stomachs. Coconut oil capsules are not only beneficial for human consumption but can also have numerous benefits for pets. The natural fats in coconut oil can help improve the coat and skin of dogs and cats, making it a popular addition to their diet. It is also believed to boost their immune system, improve their digestion, and even reduce bad breath. Just like humans, pets can consume coconut oil capsules directly or have it mixed with their food. When purchasing coconut oil capsules, it is essential to choose a reputable brand that uses high-quality, organic coconut oil. This ensures that one is getting a pure and potent form of coconut oil without any harmful additives. The dosage of the capsules may vary depending on the brand, but it is generally recommended to start with a small amount and gradually increase it to avoid any adverse reactions.

coconut oil benefit

1. Boosts Immune System Coconut oil is rich in lauric acid, a medium-chain fatty acid that is known for its antiviral, antibacterial, and antifungal properties. When consumed, lauric acid is converted into monolaurin, a compound that helps to fight off harmful pathogens in the body. This makes coconut oil an effective immune booster that can protect you against infections and illnesses. 2. Promotes Heart Health

Despite being a saturated fat, coconut oil has been shown to have a positive impact on heart health. Studies have found that the medium-chain fatty acids in coconut oil can help to increase the levels of beneficial cholesterol (HDL) while reducing the levels of harmful cholesterol (LDL). This helps to maintain a healthy balance of cholesterol in the body, reducing the risk of heart disease. 3. Supports Weight Loss The medium-chain triglycerides (MCTs) found in coconut oil are easily digested and converted into energy, making it a great source of fuel for the body. Unlike long-chain fatty acids, MCTs are not stored in the body as fat, but instead, are used as immediate energy. This can help to boost metabolism and aid in weight loss. Additionally, coconut oil has been found to help reduce appetite and cravings, making it easier to stick to a healthy diet. 4. Improves Digestive Health Coconut oil contains a significant amount of antifungal and antibacterial properties that can help to eliminate harmful bacteria in the gut. This, in turn, can improve overall digestive health and reduce the risk of digestive issues such as bloating, constipation, and irritable bowel syndrome (IBS). It has also been found to be beneficial for those with inflammatory bowel diseases such as Crohn's and ulcerative colitis. 5. Protects Skin and Hair Coconut oil is a common ingredient in skincare and haircare products due to its moisturizing, anti-inflammatory, and antimicrobial properties. It can help to hydrate and nourish the skin, reducing dryness and preventing premature aging. It can also soothe skin conditions such as eczema, psoriasis, and dermatitis. When used on the hair, coconut oil can help to repair damage, promote growth, and combat dandruff and scalp infections. 6. Balances Hormones Hormonal imbalances can lead to a range of health issues, including irregular periods, acne, weight gain, and mood swings. Consuming coconut oil has been found to help balance hormones due to its anti-inflammatory, antioxidant, and hormone-regulating properties. It can also help to improve insulin sensitivity, which is important for those with diabetes or PCOS. 7. Alleviates Inflammation Inflammation is the body's natural response to injury or infection. However, chronic inflammation has been linked to various diseases, including arthritis, heart disease, and cancer. The anti-inflammatory compounds in coconut oil can help to alleviate inflammation and reduce the risk of chronic disease. It has also been found to be effective in reducing symptoms of arthritis and other inflammatory conditions. 8. Regulates Blood Sugar Levels Research has shown that the medium-chain fatty acids in coconut oil can improve insulin sensitivity and help regulate blood sugar levels. This makes it a suitable dietary supplement for those with diabetes or at risk of developing the disease. It can also help to prevent insulin resistance, a condition that can lead to type 2 diabetes. 9. Anti-Cancer Properties While more research is needed, preliminary studies have shown that the lauric acid in coconut oil has anti-cancer properties. It has been found to be effective against cancer cells in the lab and may also help to reduce the risk of developing certain types of cancer, such as breast and colon cancer. The antioxidants in coconut oil may also play a role in protecting against cancer by reducing oxidative stress and inflammation in the body. 10. Aids in Brain Function The brain relies on glucose for energy, but when glucose levels are low, the brain can use ketones as an alternative source of fuel. The medium-chain fatty acids in coconut oil can be converted into ketones, making it a great source of energy for the brain. This can help to improve cognitive function, memory, and focus, making coconut oil beneficial for those with Alzheimer's and other neurological disorders.

The end

www.ingramcontent.com/pod-product-compliance
Lightning Source LLC
Chambersburg PA
CBHW051927250726
48659CB00002B/877